My Breastfeedir

An interactive guide

What is this book and how should I use it?

This book has been designed by an infant feeding expert to help you set and smash your lactation goals. Whether you want to provide one colostrum feed via a syringe, breastfeed to natural term, pump, combi feed, overcome challenges, or wean as soon as possible, this book will act as a prompt, a support, and a companion throughout your breastfeeding journey and beyond.

The first section of this book has several interactive worksheets covering the perinatal period. It then has a section of lined paper which you can use as a journal, for record keeping, or anything else. Finally, the end of the book has more worksheets – this time to help you as you come to the end of your breastfeeding journey.

The information in this book is evidence based as of 2022. However, it should act as a general guide and not as a replacement for medical advice or individualised care.

Our journey...

_____

And baby

_____

Born on:

_____

Part One: The Perinatal Period
Information to help you design your postnatal plan

Before your baby is born:
You have probably already come across the idea of a birth plan, but have you thought about a breastfeeding plan? Coming up with some preferences can be helpful for the people supporting you in the hours and days after baby is born and you may be surprised to know that there are several areas where you can make choices regarding feeding your baby. It's not as simple as breast or bottle! Use the following information to help you decide how to fill out the postnatal plan on the next pages:

The Golden Hour
- If your baby is born full term and healthy, you do not have to be separated initially – even to have baby weighed. Removing baby from your chest to weigh them may interrupt the process which leads to the first breastfeed and cause some degree of stress to your new baby.
- Usually any routine procedures, including weighing, can happen AFTER the first breastfeed.
- Equally, if you DO want to have baby weighed ASAP, or if you need to be separated for any reason – you can recreate the Golden Hour, even weeks later.

Hands on, or hands off?
- Generally, it is understood that allowing you and baby to figure out the first feed alone can help you to feel more confident going forward, and may help baby to latch better right from the start.
- However, if there are any concerns about you or your baby, the first feed may need to happen a bit faster.
- If you're feeling really unsure about how to breastfeed, having someone latch baby for you might help you to see and feel what's needed.
- If you then can't latch baby yourself, you may feel as though there is something wrong with you – knocking your confidence.
- You can ask for the SORT of help that feels right for you. Hands ON, is where a midwife will latch baby for you. Hands OFF is where they will demonstrate and talk you through how to latch baby, but not touch either of you.

If you are too unwell to breastfeed:
- You can give consent before birth for someone to express milk for you if you are too unwell to do this yourself.
- You could hand express before the baby is born and request that this is given if any supplements needed while you are unable to express.
- You could allow your baby to have formula until you are well enough to express or breastfeed.
- A combination of all of the above!

If your baby is too unwell to breastfeed:
- You can request that only your expressed milk is provided.
- You can discuss with peers about informal donor milk if this feels appropriate.
- You can give permission for formula to make up any deficit.

If Top-Ups are recommended:
- These can be your pumped milk
- In the first month, use the calculation 150 - 200ml per kg per day to check that the amount advised is accurate. (Example. Your baby is 3kgs. They need 150ml of milk per KG per day. 150ml x 3 = 450ml of milk daily. If your baby feeds 10x a day, that's 45ml per feed. This would be for a baby ONLY having expressed milk or formula. YOUR baby is taking some milk from the breast so less top up is likely needed.)
- Seek EXPERT support to help protect your milk supply and baby's breastfeeding instincts.

Who are the experts:

- ## Infant Feeding Support Worker
This is someone who works in your local community. In the UK they are employed by the NHS or your local infant feeding project. Their training varies, but you can expect a minimum of several hours with annual updates. Typically people in this role are passionate about infant feeding.

- ## Breastfeeding Counsellor
A parent who has breastfed – usually for at least 6 months, but requirements vary depending on the organisation they have trained with. Breastfeeding Counsellors undergo around 2 years of training and use information and active listening skills to help you problem solve, reflect, and reach your individual goals. Annual update training is usually required for a breastfeeding counsellor.

- **IBCLC (International Board Certified Lactation Consultant.)**

A health professional with a globally recognised qualification. An IBCLC must have a minimum of 1000 hours of active experience supporting breastfeeding, 90 hours of breastfeeding specific education, and then sit a two hour examination. In addition to this they must either be qualified as a health professional (nurse, Dr etc) or undergo numerous health science qualifications at a college level before they can apply for their exam. An IBCLC must update their certification every 5 years, either by sitting the exam again or through evidence of continuing education and training in the form of CERPS (Continuing Education Recognition Points)

- **What about a Peer Supporter?**

I really recommend everyone attends peer support groups. These are run by volunteers who have breastfed and then had some training to allow them to support other parents. The training varies, but typically includes how to help with basic latching, recognising the signs that you may need to see a DR, self-care tips for issues such as blocked ducts, and active listening skills. Peer supporters are often not experts, but they ARE knowledgeable, excellent at knowing when you need to see someone else, are passionate about breastfeeding, often feel called to volunteer because they struggled with breastfeeding and want to help others, make an excellent cup of tea, feed you biscuits and cake, and have fantastic listening skills. A peer support group is a fantastic starting point for seeking help. Often it is the only place you need to go, but if you do need something more – they'll tell you and help you to find that extra support.

On the next page is a one page plan you can share with your birth team. This plan covers the first hours after birth and is simple and clear.

FURTHER READING FOR THIS SECTION

Delayed weighing / Golden Hour: Crenshaw J. T. (2014). Healthy Birth Practice #6: Keep Mother and Baby Together- It's Best for Mother, Baby, and Breastfeeding. The Journal of perinatal education, 23(4), 211–217. https://doi.org/10.1891/1058-1243.23.4.211

Informal milk sharing: https://www.eatsonfeets.org/safeMilkSharing

150ml per kg per day: Maintaining milk supply as the baby grows. (2018). Australian prescriber, 41(3), 64–65. https://doi.org/10.18773/austprescr.2018.027

FEEDING OUR BABY

Human Milk feeding is important to us. Please take note of these preferences to help all of us work together in regard to feeding our baby.

The Golden Hour:

Please weigh my baby before / after our first breastfeed

Please do / do not offer hands on help with feeding

I do / do not want my baby to breast crawl

If I am too unwell to breastfeed my baby:

I do / do not give permission for someone to express my milk if I am unconsious

Please feed my baby with a cup / syringe / bottle if I am unable to breastfeed

If my baby is unable to breastfeed:

I do / do not need help with hand expressing

I do / do not consent to formula being given prior to discussion with myself.

Please do / do not give my baby a pacifier if in NICU

If top ups are needed:

I would prefer to use my expressed milk / formula in the first instance

I would prefer to use a cup / syringe / bottle

I would prefer to give LESS top up and have more frequent weight checks / I would prefer to give MORE top ups and have less frequent weight checks

I do / do not need help with a pumping plan

Our Team:

IBCLC Name and Number:

Local Peer Support Group meeting details:

Local Breastfeeding Counsellor:

Tongue tie provider:

Antenatal Hand Expression

Antenatal hand expression is where you collect colostrum in the last weeks of your pregnancy and then freeze it so that if your baby needs a top up in the days after they are born, you already have some milk ready for them. This can be especially helpful if you're anxious that you might struggle to breastfeed or if there's a chance you or baby might be unwell after the birth.

Things to consider:
- Antenatal hand expression should only be done from around 36 weeks of pregnancy and only if your care provider tells you it's safe to do so.
- Not everyone can hand express. If you don't get any milk this is NOT a sign that you won't be able to breastfeed!
- You must make sure you practice good hygiene when hand expressing – wash your hands and use new syringes to collect the milk.
- It is NORMAL to only see tiny drops of milk – a 1ml syringe is recommended for this reason!
- The average newborn needs 5ml of milk per feed on day one of their life. You don't need to express lots!

How to Hand Express:
- Firstly, wash your hands well.
- Have your 1ml syringe open and ready to draw up any drops you produce.
- Many people find gently massaging and squeezing the breast helps to get more milk.
- Use your fingers and thumb to make a C shape around your breast near the edge of your areola.
- Push your fingers and thumb backwards towards your chest.
- Squeeze your fingers and thumbs gently together.
- Release the pressure, keeping your hand around the breast.
- Repeat!
- When you see a drop of colostrum draw it up into the syringe.
- When you have finished, secure a cap on the syringe, use a label to date the milk, and then put it in a Ziploc bag in the freezer.
- There are many great videos online where you can see someone hand expressing in real time. This can help you to understand the technique better.

FURTHER READING FOR THIS SECTION

Demirci, J. R., Glasser, M., Fichner, J., Caplan, E., & Himes, K. P. (2019). "It gave me so much confidence": First-time U.S. mothers' experiences with antenatal milk expression. Maternal & child nutrition, 15(4), e12824.
https://doi.org/10.1111/mcn.12824

My colostrum harvesting record:

Date: Time: Amount:

Notes:
(Technique, any preparation steps that helped, how you're feeling...)

Date: Time: Amount:

Notes:
(Technique, any preparation steps that helped, how you're feeling...)

Date: Time: Amount:

Notes:
(Technique, any preparation steps that helped, how you're feeling...)

Date: Time: Amount:

Notes:
(Technique, any preparation steps that helped, how you're feeling...)

My colostrum harvesting record:

Date: Time: Amount:

Notes:
(Technique, any preparation steps that helped, how you're feeling...)

Date: Time: Amount:

Notes:
(Technique, any preparation steps that helped, how you're feeling...)

Date: Time: Amount:

Notes:
(Technique, any preparation steps that helped, how you're feeling...)

Date: Time: Amount:

Notes:
(Technique, any preparation steps that helped, how you're feeling...)

My colostrum harvesting record:

Date: Time: Amount:

Notes:
(Technique, any preparation steps that helped, how you're feeling...)

Date: Time: Amount:

Notes:
(Technique, any preparation steps that helped, how you're feeling...)

Date: Time: Amount:

Notes:
(Technique, any preparation steps that helped, how you're feeling...)

Date: Time: Amount:

Notes:
(Technique, any preparation steps that helped, how you're feeling...)

Why Breastfeed?

There are many reasons why breastfeeding is great for your baby, you, and the planet! It
Can you find some information in a breastfeeding book or online to help you fill in this
section?

Why is breastfeeding important to me?

How breastfeeding helps my baby:

How breastfeeding helps my health:

How breastfeeding helps the planet:

How breastfeeding helps my daily life:

Our first breastfeed:

Day: Time: Place:

Everything I remember:

_____

_____

_____

_____

_____

_____

_____

_____

_____

_____

_____

A photo

Signs Feeding Is Going Well

In the first 24hrs after baby is born you should see them pass their sticky meconium poo. They should then poo DAILY until around week 6. There is a common misconception, even among some health professionals, that breastfed babies don't poo daily because of how efficient human milk is. This is NOT TRUE in the first 6 weeks of life. Lack of dirty nappies during this time often suggests that baby is not getting as much milk as they need, or that they may have a problem with their tummy.

You should also see ONE wet nappy (or more) per day of life until your milk supply becomes abundant around days 3 – 5. Eg: one nappy on day one, 2 on day two etc.

After your milk "comes in" you should notice around 6 heavy wet nappies per day. Urine should be light in colour and not smell strongly of ammonia.

Use the chart below to keep on track of the minimum output expected for each of the first five days:

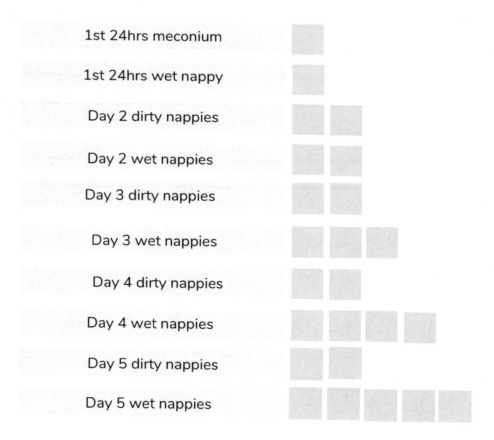

1st 24hrs meconium

1st 24hrs wet nappy

Day 2 dirty nappies

Day 2 wet nappies

Day 3 dirty nappies

Day 3 wet nappies

Day 4 dirty nappies

Day 4 wet nappies

Day 5 dirty nappies

Day 5 wet nappies

FURTHER READING FOR THIS SECTION

https://www.nct.org.uk/baby-toddler/nappies-and-poo/newborn-baby-poo-nappies-what-expect

https://breastfeedingusa.org/content/article/diaper-output-and-milk-intake-early-weeks

Other signs that feeding is going well:

- ## You are in a comfortable position
This means that you are less likely to move and accidentally change baby's latch. It will also reduce the risk of muscular pain and help your baby to get a deeper latch because they will sense that your muscles are relaxed.

- ## Baby's front is touching your body
Babies need to feel grounded and safe to breastfeed. Providing them with as much physical contact as possible can help to achieve this. It also ensures baby is as close to you as possible, which will help wit achieving a deep latch as baby won't have to stretch to feed.

- ## Nose to nipple
When you line up baby's nose to your nipple for feeding, rather than pointing your nipple at their mouth, baby will tip their head back and take a deeper mouthful of breast.

- ## Feeding is not painful for you
Pain tells us that your nipple is in the wrong part of baby's mouth, and that means that baby won't be removing milk as well as they could be.

- ## Baby is swallowing
Listen for a "keh" sound and look for deep jaw movements. When your milk is flowing fast you can expect there to be rhythmic, frequent swallows. It is normal for baby to slow down, and then speed up again, usually finishing the feed with sporadic swallowing.

- ## Baby is relaxed or sleepy after feeding
A baby who is crying after feeding is usually still hungry, or uncomfortable.

- ## Your nipple is rounded after feeds
If your nipple is pinched, squashed, slanted or a different colour to usual after feeds this suggests it wasn't far enough back in baby's mouth, and that baby was probably not removing milk as well as they could be.

- ## Wet nappies
If it's going in, it's got to come out! If you are not seeing frequent, light coloured nappies your baby may be dehydrated.

- ## Dirty nappies
In the first 6 weeks, your milk is high in whey protein. This "whizzes" through the digestive system and it is normal for you to see some poo at most feeds. You should see AT LEAST two dirty nappies a day, and the poo should be the size of an "ok" sign you make with your thumb and finger.

- **Feeding 8-12 times per 24 hour period**

Less than 8 feeds a day suggest baby may be too sleepy or weak to take milk. More than 12 feeds can be normal, but it depends on all of the other things you're seeing. If baby is growing well, producing lots of nappies, relaxed after feeds, and you are not in pain then feeding more than 12x is likely for comfort, pain relief, reassurance and sleep support. (all normal and all totally ok to allow!)

The good feed checklist:

What you're looking for:	✓	✗
You are in a comfortable position		
Your baby has their front touching your body		
Nose to nipple!		
Feeding is not painful for you		
You can see baby is swallowing		
Baby's chin is touching the breast		
Your nipple is rounded after feeds		
Baby is producing wet nappies		
Baby is producing dirty nappies		
8 - 12 feeds per 24 hours		
ACTIVE feeding lasts at least 5 minutes		
Feeding takes less than an hour		
Baby is sleepy / relaxed after feeding		

When the days are long...

I can ask these people for support:

These are the places I can go for fresh air:

These are the TV shows/audiobooks/podcasts I want to catch up on:

Easy to prepare foods I enjoy are:

When the nights are long...

Safe Sleep 7

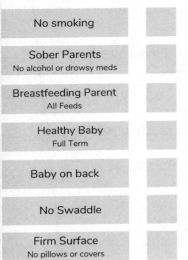

No smoking	
Sober Parents No alcohol or drowsy meds	
Breastfeeding Parent All Feeds	
Healthy Baby Full Term	
Baby on back	
No Swaddle	
Firm Surface No pillows or covers	

We understand that following these guidelines for bed-sharing may reduce the risk of sudden infant death syndrome. Most cases of SIDS happen when the parent accidentally falls asleep with their baby in an unprepared environment or on a sofa.

However, the discussion for safe sleep is a big one so please make full use of wider resources to help inform your decision:
- Basis online
- Lullaby Trust
- LLL Safe Sleep 7

This document only gives an overview of bed-sharing guidance. It is your responsibility to research and make appropriate decisions for your family set up.

And things feel really tough...

Midnight snacks to keep me going:

Online communities where people are awake:

My plan for when I'm too tired:

Seeking More Help

This UK sources are reputable and can help you with many challenges.

Lactation Consultants of Great Britain (Find an IBCLC)
https://lcgb.org/find-an-ibclc/

Association of Tongue Tie Providers (Find a tongue tie provider)
https://www.tongue-tie.org.uk/find-a-practitioner/

National Breastfeeding Helpline 0300 100 0212
https://www.nationalbreastfeedinghelpline.org.uk/

LLL helpline 0345 120 2918
https://www.laleche.org.uk/telephone-helpline/

NCT helpline 0300 330 0700
https://www.nct.org.uk/baby-toddler/feeding/early-days/support-breastfeeding-or-bottle-feeding-our-infant-feeding-line

LLL website
https://www.laleche.org.uk/

Drugs in breastmilk information service
https://www.breastfeedingnetwork.org.uk/detailed-information/drugs-in-breastmilk/

Reflecting on week one:

The highlights

The challenges

Things to work on

I'm most proud of...

Troubleshooting

It's very common to have worries and problems in the first few weeks of breastfeeding. These pages will help you to figure out if you're experiencing something "normal" or if you might need some more help.

Weight Loss

In the first 5 days of life it is normal for babies to lose 5-7% of their birth weight, and common for them to lose up to 10%. If your baby has lost MORE than 10% of their birth weight on day 5, or if they are not beginning to regain their lost weight by days 7 – 10, OR if they are not close to birth weight by day 14 then this suggests that further help is needed.

Nappies

As already discussed, if it's coming out... it's going in! We want to see a **MINIMUM** of 2 dirty nappies per 24 hours and around 6 **HEAVY** wet nappies per 24 hours.

Your Comfort

If breastfeeding is painful for you something is wrong. It is likely that your baby isn't latching as well as they need to in order to remove as much milk as possible. This can lead to more frequent feeding, slow weight gain, and fussiness.

Alert and Relaxed Periods

A newborn baby will take some time each day to quietly observe the world. If they are not doing this because they are always crying or sleeping, you may have a feeding issue.

Waking for Feeds

A baby that does not wake for feeds may be too weak to wake up due to struggling to take enough milk.

FURTHER READING FOR THIS SECTION

https://cks.nice.org.uk/topics/faltering-growth/management/weight-loss-in-the-first-few-days-after-birth/

https://www.unicef.org.uk/babyfriendly/baby-friendly-resources/implementing-standards-resources/breastfeeding-assessment-tools/

Frequent Feeding

It is very normal for a baby to feed between 8 and 12 times a day, and sometimes more. However, there is a bigger picture we need to consider. Use this checklist to reassure you, or as an outline to ask for further support.

	✓	✗
My baby has lost less than 10% of their birth weight		
My baby is starting to gain weight		
I'm seeing at least 2 dirty nappies a day		
I'm seeing about 6 wet nappies a day		
Breastfeeding is not painful for me		
There are times each day where my baby seems alert and calm		
My baby wakes for feeds		

If you have ticked "no" to any of these, you may want to seek extra help from an IBCLC, breastfeeding counsellor, infant feeding support worker, or a helpline.

Topping Up

Hearing that you need to top up can be upsetting, but it's very common as you and baby learn how to feed. Assuming your long term goal is to exclusively breastfeed, the following list can help you to talk to your care provider about how to make sure you have a robust plan in place. There's also a feeding plan template you can use, and a record chart to document all the essentials while you're working on getting things back on track.

Please note that the information on the following pages is only a guide. It is VERY important that you work with your Health Care Provider to ensure your baby's individual needs are met.

Questions to ask your care provider before topping up:

What specific concerns do you currently have about my baby's health?

Have you observed my baby swallowing well at the breast?

Do you have any techniques we can try to improve at breast feeding? If not, can you refer me to someone who does?

What other options do we have today?

How have you worked out the volume of top up you're recommending?

When will you reassess the plan?

What can I use instead of a bottle?

Could there be a tongue tie?

This information acts as a guide. Please work with your Health Care Provider to help you decide how much milk your baby needs.

How much milk does my baby need?

Day 1
5-7ml per feed

Day 3
18 - 30ml per feed

Day 7
45-60ml per feed

After one week:

150-200ml per kg of body weight, per day.

Example: a 3kg baby needs 450 - 600ml of milk per day.

Divide this total by the number of feeds to work out per feed amount.

EG - 8 feeds for a 3kg baby would be 56 - 75ml per feed.
(450 or 600 divided by 8)

After one month:

750 - 1000ml per day, with an average of 900ml per day.

Working out top ups:

Work out how much your baby SHOULD weigh:

Average gain after week 1 is 25 - 30g per day

A baby who weighs 3kgs on day 10 should gain 75-90g in the next 72hrs.

If they gain 35g we can guess they need about 50% top ups.

Full volume would be around 450ml, so divide this in half to work out daily top ups needed.

In this case it is 225ml. Divide this by 8 to find your per feed volume. Here, it is 28ml

Topping up plan:

Date started:

Today's weight:

Date of re-assessment:

Ideal weight:

Give   ml of EBM / Formula   times per day.

Top up method:

Cup / syringe / bottle / tube

Pumping routine:

(Ideally pump for 10 - 20 minutes for each top up given)

Evaluation:

How much has baby gained?

Recalculated top up volume:

Weight goal:

Goal Date:

Important note: You should work with a health care provider to help you decide the best plan for you and your baby.

Top up Methods

Syringe

Useful for small volumes.
Quick and easy.
Risk of aspiration.
Risk of baby developing preference.

Our notes on this method

Cup

Cheap and easy to clean.
Helps with tongue movements.
Slow and messy.

Our notes on this method

Bottle

Socially normal
Easy to use
Can lead to bottle preference

Our notes on this method

Tube at breast

Avoids supplements away from the breast
May support milk supply
Can help baby learn to breastfeed
Hard to access
Complicated to clean

Our notes on this method

More information

Syringe feeding
https://www.youtube.com/watch?v=d4KQULz9u5Q

Cup feeding
https://www.youtube.com/watch?v=X2t57eNGMEs&t=29s

Paced bottle feeding
https://www.youtube.com/watch?v=TuZXD1hIW8Q&t=9s

At breast tube supplementing
https://www.youtube.com/watch?v=gRCitroQDvk

In depth article for slow weight gain
https://breastfeeding.support/supplementing-an-underweight-baby/

Input and output record

Date:

Time	Breastfed	Top up volume	Amount pumped	Wet / dirty nappy
Time				
Time				
Time				
Time				
Time				
Time				
Time				
Time				
Time				
Time				
Time				
Time				
Time				
Time				

Input and output record

Date:

Time	Breastfed	Top up volume	Amount pumped	Wet / dirty nappy
Time				
Time				
Time				
Time				
Time				
Time				
Time				
Time				
Time				
Time				
Time				
Time				
Time				
Time				

Input and output record

Date:

Time	Breastfed	Top up volume	Amount pumped	Wet / dirty nappy
Time				
Time				
Time				
Time				
Time				
Time				
Time				
Time				
Time				
Time				
Time				
Time				
Time				
Time				

Input and output record

Date:

Time	Breastfed	Top up volume	Amount pumped	Wet / dirty nappy
Time				
Time				
Time				
Time				
Time				
Time				
Time				
Time				
Time				
Time				
Time				
Time				
Time				
Time				

Input and output record

Date:

Time	Breastfed	Top up volume	Amount pumped	Wet / dirty nappy
Time				
Time				
Time				
Time				
Time				
Time				
Time				
Time				
Time				
Time				
Time				
Time				
Time				
Time				

Milestones in the First Weeks

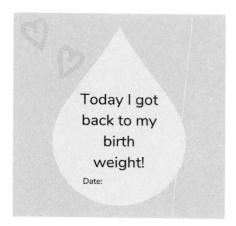

Today I got back to my birth weight!

Date:

Today we saw a Lactation Consultant!

Date:

We went to the breastfeeding support group for the first time!

Date:

I visited the osteopath!

Date:

Discharged from the midwives!

Date:

I gained this much weight!

_____

Date:

Reflecting on week 2

What went well

What was challenging

What we need to work on next week

What I'm most proud of

Growth Spurts

In the early days and weeks of life babies frequently have days where they want to feed more often than usual, and may be fussy. This can happen around the clock, not just in the day. Growth spurt behaviour can be worrying, so this check list can help you to decide if there is something else happening.

Probably normal

Around 6 heavy wet nappies per 24hrs	
Yellow, seedy nappies at least 2x daily	
Behaviour is new / you've had a period of easier feeds	
Weight gain has been on track	
Breastfeeding is not painful for you	
Baby appears healthy	

Seek extra help
(From a Health Care Provider)

Less wet nappies than usual	
Less dirty nappies than usual	
Dirty nappies are green or have mucous in them	
Any other strange colour of poop	
You are in pain	
Baby appears unwell in ANY way	

Is frequent feeding normal during growth spurts?

Yes! During a period of rapid development your baby is learning many new things, and using more energy than usual. Your body will make more milk when baby feeds more often. This is why we often describe breastfeeding as DEMAND and SUPPLY (not supply and demand.) It is not uncommon for babies to want to feed very often for a day or two during a growth spurt. They may also be fussy during this period. Remembering to look at the basics for good feeding can help to reassure you, or help you to decide to seek more help if needed.

More Reading

https://kellymom.com/hot-topics/growth-spurts/

Reflecting on week 3

What went well

What was challenging

What we need to work on next week

What I'm most proud of

Reflecting on week 4

What went well

What was challenging

What we need to work on next week

What I'm most proud of

Common Hurdles - Pain

Pain can come up even after you've overcome your very early challenges. While positioning and attachment (including issues caused by tongue tie) remains the most common cause of pain, it's also a good idea to know about thrush and mastitis:

Why am I in pain?

Thrush checklist:

Pain in both breasts / nipples	
Pain is new	
Nipples are itchy / burning	
Pain is worse after feeds	
Baby has a nappy rash	
New clicking / fussing at breast	

Next Steps:

1. See your GP for a swab and treatment if indicated.

2. BOTH Mum AND baby MUST be treated.

3. Wash any clothing that has been in contact with your breasts on a hot (60c) wash and line dry outside if possible.

4. Wash and teething toys / bottles / dummies with sterilising solution, in the dishwasher, or by boiling.

See The Drugs in Breastmilk Information Service Factsheet for Thrush for more details.

Mastitis Checklist

One sided pain	
Bruised feeling in the breast	
Redness / darker patch of skin (depending on skin colour.)	
Fever / Flu type symptoms	
Breast fullness even after feeding	

Next Steps:

1. Keep breastfeeding or pumping

2. See your Dr for diagnosis and treatment if needed.

3. Massage the breast before and during feeds to help remove milk

4. Apply heat before feeds to open milk ducts

5. Use ibuprofen / paracetamol as appropriate for you personally

See Kellmom.com article called "Plugged Ducts and Mastitis" for more info

Important note on blocked ducts

Blocked ducts and mastitis have many similar symptoms. If you do not have a fever or feel unwell, feeding is tolerable and baby is happy you might want to use self care measures for up to 73 hours before seeking medical advice. However, if you are in doubt AT ALL it is best to talk to your DR.

Part Two: The Journal

The following pages are simply blank. You might want to use them to document your breastfeeding journey, to record pumping or nappy output, or to just doodle. There is no right or wrong way to use them. At the end you will find a final section of worksheets to help you process the end of your breastfeeding journey – whenever that happens to be.

Part Three: Ending Your Journey

Whether it's a week, a month, or several years; when the time comes to end breastfeeding you may experience a range of feelings. It's normal to feel sad, worried, lost, or even angry depending on how you have reached this point. These last pages of worksheets can help you to process your experience, mark it and close this chapter of parenting with pride and satisfaction.

Am I ready to stop?

When I think about no longer breastfeeding, I feel the benefits are...

When I think about no longer breastfeeding, the worries I have are...

My notes on the weaning methods I have come across and how they feel to me:

How it started...	How it ended...
Photo	Photo

The challenges we overcame

The most unusual place we fed

My favourite memory of breastfeeding

Our word for feeding:	Total number of days we fed:

Our weaning plan

Start date:

Planned date of last feed:

Step one:

Step two:

Step three:

If it feels overwhelming we will...

What has my experience of breastfeeding taught me?

If You Stopped Before You Wanted To

Breastfeeding doesn't always go to plan and sometimes it just doesn't work in the way you had hoped. If you stop breastfeeding before you wanted to it's very common to feel guilt, shame, confusion, or anger. However, it is important to understand that the system in the West is set up to fail mothers – you are NOT at fault. The support that parents have access to is inconsistent and often lacking due to staff shortages, limited training, and formula feeding being normal in our culture. If we lived in a breastfeeding friendly culture, everyone who has contact with new parents would know how to support breastfeeding appropriately. The fact that we need to seek out specialist lactation care in the West tells us that it is not a priority for those in charge.

You can seek a "debrief" for your breastfeeding experience. This is where a breastfeeding counsellor, IBCLC, doula, or similar will sit with you and hold space while you recount your story. This person will often help you to see where the system failed you as a way of helping you to reframe your experience. The following worksheet can act as a starting point, or a basic "self-help" debrief but it doesn't replace expert support.

Processing my experience

What went wrong:

How I feel about it:

What I know about it now:

The support and information I should have had but didn't:

What I want to say to those who let us down:

What I would do differently next time:

I'm proud that...

Away from breastfeeding, I connect with my baby by:

My baby loves it when I...

Thank you for using this guide!

Lucy has already had two books published by Praeclarus Press - Relactation and Mixed Up.
Her next book, Breastfeeding Myths is due to be released on July 15th 2022

You can find Lucy on Facebook and Instagram, or at
lucyruddle_ibclc@outlook.com

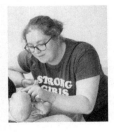
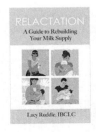
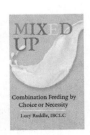
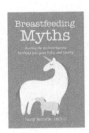

Printed in Great Britain
by Amazon

27421217R00057